I0697456

BATTLING FIBROMYALGIA

Comprehensive Guide To Understanding, Managing, Thriving & Pathways To Recovery

ROGER ANDREW

© 2023 By Roger Andrew

All Rights Reserved.

It is important to note that without the publisher's express written permission, you may not copy, distribute, or transmit any part of this publication in any form, including but not limited to electronic or mechanical reproduction or transmission. It is important to note that this limitation may not apply to brief quotations that are incorporated into critical evaluations and certain noncommercial applications permitted by copyright law.

Contents

Introductory

Pain that radiates throughout the body, discomfort in the muscles and other soft tissues, and other symptoms are hallmarks of the chronic medical illness known as fibromyalgia. The precise mechanism by which it causes an abnormally high pain threshold and heightened pain response is yet unknown, however it is thought to involve abnormalities in the brain and spinal cord.

Fibromyalgia is characterized by the following symptoms and signs:

• Pain That Is Pervasive Fibromyalgia sufferers often report experiencing pain on both sides of their bodies and above and below the waist. The pain is commonly described as a dull, continuous ache, but it can sometimes be sharp and severe.

• Specific painful sites on the body are often used to diagnose fibromyalgia. There are certain spots that are extremely tender to the touch and can cause severe discomfort.

• Sleep disturbances: People with fibromyalgia generally have trouble going asleep, wake up frequently throughout the night, and have trouble getting back to sleep.

• Problems with Thinking: People with fibromyalgia sometimes suffer from what is called "fibro fog," which can make it hard for them to focus, remember details, and think clearly.

• Morning stiffness is a frequent symptom of fibromyalgia and can make it difficult to get up and moving first thing in the morning.

• Headaches, Irritable Bowel Syndrome (IBS), Depression, Anxiety, and Neuropathic Pain or Numbness in the Hands and Feet May Also Be Associated with Fibromyalgia.

Due to the lack of diagnostic laboratory testing or imaging studies, the diagnosis of fibromyalgia is frequently determined by a process of exclusion. The diagnostic process is further complicated by the fact that it might coexist with other medical disorders.

Medication (including analgesics, antidepressants, and anti-seizure medications), physical therapy, exercise, stress management, and dietary and lifestyle changes may all play a role in the treatment of fibromyalgia.

Fibromyalgia patients should collaborate closely with their doctors to create a treatment plan that is unique to their condition and symptoms.

CHAPTER ONE
Diagnosis Methods

Since there are currently no confirmed diagnostic laboratory testing or imaging investigations for fibromyalgia, the diagnostic process might be lengthy. Instead, a healthcare provider will conduct a thorough evaluation to rule out other potential causes of the patient's symptoms before making a diagnosis of fibromyalgia. The diagnostic procedure consists of the following steps:

• First, your doctor will take a thorough medical history by asking you questions about your symptoms, how long they've lasted, what might have triggered them, and any other health issues that might be relevant. It is also helpful to share details about your family's health history.

• You'll get checked out physically to see how you're doing generally and pinpoint any trouble spots in your muscles and tendons. However, the presence of tender spots is only one element of the evaluation for fibromyalgia.

• Since fibromyalgia symptoms may resemble those of other medical issues, your doctor will do their best to rule out those other conditions. It may be necessary to consider and test for conditions such rheumatoid arthritis, lupus, thyroid disorders, and multiple sclerosis.

• Blood tests are commonly used in the lab to examine inflammation indicators, rule out autoimmune illnesses, and evaluate thyroid health. These examinations can rule out other potential causes of the symptoms being experienced.

• To rule out structural problems or other musculoskeletal diseases, doctors may order imaging procedures like X-rays or magnetic resonance imaging (MRI).

• Criteria for Diagnosis Fibromyalgia is often diagnosed when certain conditions are met. Among the criteria defined by the American College of Rheumatology (ACR) are generalized pain and the existence of tender spots.

Recent guidelines, however, have evolved away from emphasis on tender points and instead focus on the pervasive nature of the pain and other identifying symptoms including exhaustion and sleep disruptions.

• Your doctor will evaluate the frequency and severity of symptoms like exhaustion, sleep problems, brain fog, and mood swings that are associated with fibromyalgia.

• Your primary care physician may recommend that you see a neurologist, rheumatologist, or pain management specialist for further assessment and consultation based on your symptoms and medical history.

• Once a diagnosis of fibromyalgia has been made, it is essential to collaborate with your healthcare team to develop a specialized treatment plan that takes into account your unique symptoms. Medication, physical therapy, behavioral changes, and other forms of pain management may all figure into this strategy. Improving your quality of life will require constant monitoring and the treatment of associated symptoms.

It's worth noting that diagnosing fibromyalgia can be difficult and may take some time. The diagnostic process might be made more difficult by the fact that some people with fibromyalgia also have other medical disorders.

The key to successful fibromyalgia management is creating a caring healthcare team and keeping lines of communication open with your providers.

Fibromyalgia: What We Know From Science

Fibromyalgia is a complicated and multifaceted disorder, the specific etiology of which is unknown. While research into the exact causes of fibromyalgia is ongoing, several elements and theories have been offered as possible contributors to the disorder.

Here's a rundown of everything we know about fibromyalgia now:

• Sensitization of the central nervous system is a prominent concept in the study of fibromyalgia. This hypothesis postulates that the central nervous system (CNS; think brain and spinal cord) of people with fibromyalgia reacts abnormally to pain signals. Because of this heightened sensitivity, even somewhat painless stimuli may be experienced as extremely unpleasant.

• Brains of fibromyalgia patients have been proven to process pain in an abnormal fashion, according to studies. Increased activity in brain areas responsible for pain perception and processing has been observed in people with functional MRI brain abnormalities.

• Evidence suggests that fibromyalgia may be related to neurochemical abnormalities, specifically those involving serotonin, norepinephrine, and dopamine. Mood, sleep, and the experience of pain are all influenced by these neurotransmitters. Alterations in their levels may play a role in the development of the disease.

• Fibromyalgia appears to have a genetic component, as it has a strong hereditary component. Although no one gene has been definitively linked to fibromyalgia, several genetic variants may enhance vulnerability to the disorder.

• Infections, physical or emotional trauma, and stress are all examples of environmental factors that may set off or intensify fibromyalgia symptoms in those who are prone to the disorder because of their genes.

• Poor sleep quality can exacerbate fibromyalgia symptoms, and sleep problems are prevalent with the condition. Sleep disturbances definitely have a substantial impact in the severity of fibromyalgia symptoms, while it is unclear whether they are a cause or a consequence of the condition.

• Fibromyalgia has been linked to hormonal factors, namely hormone imbalances in the hypothalamic-pituitary-adrenal (HPA) axis. The HPA axis has a role in the stress response and is associated with altered pain and inflammatory responses.

• Some studies have found links between fibromyalgia and immune system problems. Some people with the illness have been found to have abnormally high or low amounts of certain cytokines, as well as abnormal immunological responses.

Symptoms of fibromyalgia can vary greatly from one individual to the next due to the heterogeneous nature of the disorder. Different people with fibromyalgia will experience the ailment in different ways and have different causes for their symptoms.

Fibromyalgia is a complicated disorder, making it difficult to identify a single cause or mechanism. Instead, it is believed that a number of factors, including genetic, neurological, hormonal, and environmental interactions, all play a role in the onset and maintenance of fibromyalgia symptoms. More effective treatments and a deeper comprehension of the underlying mechanisms that cause the illness are the focus of ongoing research.

CHAPTER TWO
Causes Of A Flare-Up

The terms "triggers" and "flare-ups" are used interchangeably to describe the brief worsening of pain and other symptoms in people with fibromyalgia.

Chronic and widespread pain is a hallmark of fibromyalgia, but it can be exacerbated or triggered by a number of other reasons. Fibromyalgia sufferers would do well to learn to recognize and control their condition's aggravating factors.

Here are some typical causes of stress and advice for coping with them:

• Fibromyalgia symptoms can be made worse by prolonged exposure to high levels of stress. Mindfulness meditation, deep breathing exercises, and progressive muscle relaxation are just few of the stress-reduction methods that have shown promise for effective stress management.

• Overdoing it on the fitness or activity front can bring on a fibromyalgia flare-up. Pace yourself and do light workouts like swimming, walking, or yoga on a regular basis.

• Inadequate or poor quality sleep has been linked to an increase in fibromyalgia symptoms. You can get better sleep by sticking to a regular sleep schedule, making your bedroom a relaxing place, and practicing proper sleep hygiene.

• Some people with fibromyalgia report increased pain after exposure to cold or damp weather. Avoiding this set off by being warm and dressed correctly for the conditions.

• Some fibromyalgia sufferers report relief from their symptoms when their menstrual or menopausal cycles return to normal. Medications or hormone replacement treatment may be recommended by a doctor.

• Diet: Symptoms may be triggered or made worse by certain meals or dietary practices. Those who suffer from fibromyalgia may have an intolerance to processed foods, artificial sweeteners, and caffeine. A healthy lifestyle includes eating well and drinking enough of water.

• Anxiety and despair, for example, have been shown to exacerbate fibromyalgia symptoms. Treatment of mental illness through talk therapy, counseling, and medication (if needed) has been shown to have positive effects on physical health as well.

• Flare-ups of fibromyalgia can be brought on by viral infections or other disorders. Infections can be avoided by being hygienic and by getting vaccinated when necessary.

• Pollen and dust mite allergies, for example, have been linked to an exacerbation of fibromyalgia symptoms. Lessening contact with allergens and using other methods of managing allergies can be helpful.

• The adverse effects of some drugs used to treat other ailments can actually make fibromyalgia symptoms worse. If you think your prescription dosages need to be changed, talk to your doctor.

• Symptoms of fibromyalgia can be triggered or made worse by psychological stressors such major life transitions or traumatic experiences. A person's ability to deal with emotional pressures can be improved by counseling or therapy.

• Sedentary lifestyle: Chronic inactivity has been linked to increased risk of joint pain and stiffness. Avoiding this trigger might be as simple as keeping active and flexible throughout the day.

It's crucial to keep in mind that everyone's triggers and flare-ups are unique. Identifying and controlling the unique triggers for your fibromyalgia can be accomplished through the use of a symptom journal or collaboration with a healthcare specialist. Physical, emotional, and lifestyle issues all need to be considered when developing an effective plan for controlling the illness.

Adjustments To One's Way Of Life

Modifying one's way of life is crucial in the treatment of fibromyalgia. While there is currently no treatment that will reverse the effects of this disorder, there is hope in the form of lifestyle adjustments that can help lessen its impact. Here are some ways in which fibromyalgia patients' daily lives can improve:

• Low-impact exercise on a regular basis is recommended for those with fibromyalgia. Flexibility, strength, and general health can all benefit from exercises like walking, swimming, yoga, and tai chi. You should ease into your workouts and then steadily ramp up both the intensity and time.

• Eating a healthy, varied, and balanced diet can have positive effects on many aspects of your health. Choose foods that have not been processed, like fresh produce, lean proteins, and whole grains. Some people with fibromyalgia report improvement in their condition after cutting off trigger foods like caffeine and sugar substitutes.

• Sleep Well: Make sure you're receiving the shut-eye you need. Set aside time each day to sleep, make your bedroom a relaxing place to be, and practice proper sleep hygiene.

Talking to your doctor about sleep issues can help you get the help you need.

• Managing stress is an important part of caring for someone with fibromyalgia. Include mindfulness practices, meditation, deep breathing exercises, progressive muscle relaxation, and other stress-reduction strategies in your regular routine.

• Learn to moderate yourself and refrain from overexerting oneself. Don't ignore your fatigue or discomfort signals and stop what you're doing if you reach that stage. Make chores more bearable by breaking them up into smaller chunks and taking frequent pauses.

• Some people find relief from their discomfort when they apply heat or ice to the affected area. Find out what works best for you by trying various methods, such as hot baths, heating pads, and cold packs.

• Pain in the feet and legs can be alleviated by wearing shoes with adequate arch support. If you don't have the right shoes on, your alignment and posture will suffer.

• If you do a lot of work at a desk or computer, it's important to make sure your setup is ergonomic so you don't hurt yourself. Take frequent breaks to move around and stretch, keep a healthy posture, and use an adjustable chair.

• Reducing wear and tear on your muscles and joints is one benefit of keeping your weight in check. If you need help controlling your weight, talk to your doctor or a dietician.

• Emotional support can be found in one's social network, so it's important to maintain those relationships. Think about connecting with others who understand what you're going through by attending a fibromyalgia support group.

• Cognitive Behavioral Therapy (CBT): CBT can be useful for helping people with fibromyalgia deal with pain, get better sleep, and handle stressful situations. Reframing destructive thought processes and learning new coping mechanisms are major themes.

• Regarding fibromyalgia medicine, it is important to take the pills exactly as suggested by your doctor. Medication, such as analgesics, antidepressants, or other types, may help alleviate symptoms for some people.

• Reducing or eliminating alcohol and caffeine consumption has been shown to improve sleep quality and decrease anxiety.

• Relaxation and muscle tension can both be alleviated with regular use of mild stretching exercises and relaxation techniques.

Keep in mind that these changes in lifestyle can have varying degrees of success for different people. It could take some time before you figure out which methods are most effective.

To develop a treatment strategy tailored to your unique situation and symptoms, talk to your doctor or a fibromyalgia expert. If you want to prevent feeling overwhelmed, take things slowly and practice patience.

CHAPTER THREE
Techniques For Handling Stress

Because stress can increase fibromyalgia symptoms and add to pain and discomfort, learning to manage stress is essential for people who suffer from the condition. If you suffer with fibromyalgia, you may find that the following stress-reduction strategies help:

• Meditation in the present moment, free of judgment, is what's called "mindfulness." It has been shown to promote mental health and lower stress levels. You can begin with shorter sessions of guided meditation and work up to longer ones.

• Relax your nervous system and lessen your tension with the aid of deep breathing techniques, such as diaphragmatic breathing. Do some deep breathing exercises like taking a few seconds to inhale through your nose and then slowly exhaling through your mouth.

• Tensing and then relaxing several sets of muscles is a key component of progressive muscle relaxation. Physical stress and anxiety can be alleviated using this method.

• Gentle yoga has been shown to increase flexibility, lessen stress in the muscles, and facilitate restful sleep. Do some research and find a yoga class or online video that caters to people with fibromyalgia or chronic pain.

• The martial art of Tai Chi is characterized by gentle, flowing movements and deep breathing. It has the potential to enhance equilibrium, relieve stress, and boost health and happiness.

• The term "biofeedback" refers to a specific type of training that teaches you to monitor and control your own physiological responses to stress. Stress can be mitigated by learning to regulate these responses with the help of a biofeedback therapist.

• Aromatherapy: Scents like lavender and chamomile are known to induce feelings of tranquility. If you're looking to unwind, try diffusing some essential oils or taking a deep whiff of them on their own.

• To practice guided imagery, one imagines pleasant, relaxing scenes. To unwind and feel less anxious, you can either listen to prerecorded guided imagery sessions or come up with your own.

• Keeping a journal can be a healthy outlet for releasing pent-up emotions and thoughts. Describe in writing what you went through, how you felt, and what you think triggered it. By doing so, you can better understand what causes you stress and how to cope with it.

• To de-stress and feel better emotionally, spending time with compassionate friends and family is highly recommended. Talk to them about how you're feeling and tell them about any stresses you're experiencing.

• Manage your time wisely so that you don't end up stressed out by trying to do too much. Make chores more bearable by breaking them down into smaller chunks, and give yourself time to unwind.

• Cut Back on Screen Time: Spending too much time in front of the screen, especially on social media and news sites, has been linked to increased stress. Limiting your time in front of the screen can help you avoid digital stressors and negative information.

• Stress reduction and improved disposition are two of the benefits of music therapy. Make some playlists of soothing music to listen to when you need to unwind or calm down.

• Relax and let your creative side out by doing something you love, like reading, drawing, knitting, or gardening. Participating in enjoyable activities and expressing one's creativity can relieve tension and help one feel more fulfilled.

• Consult a professional counselor or therapist who focuses on chronic pain or stress reduction. You can learn healthy coping mechanisms with the help of therapy, such as cognitive-behavioral therapy (CBT).

Keep in mind that it may take some experimenting to find the most effective methods of stress management for you.

It's important to try out different methods and modify your approach to stress management based on your unique requirements and preferences, as what works for one person may not work for another. In addition, maintaining a regular routine for stress management is essential for seeing its benefits over time.

Treatments And Medications

Fibromyalgia treatment plans typically incorporate a variety of approaches aimed at alleviating the patient's unique set of symptoms. Remember that there is no magic bullet for fibromyalgia, and that treatment methods may need to be modified as the condition progresses. The following are some of the most often prescribed drugs and treatments for fibromyalgia:

Medications:

• For moderate discomfort, your doctor may prescribe a pain medication such ibuprofen or acetaminophen, both of which are available without a prescription. However, these are typically not helpful for the discomfort associated with fibromyalgia.

• Pain relievers available by prescription include opioid analgesics and tramadol for moderate to severe pain. Because of their addictive qualities and negative side effects, opioids are rarely used unless absolutely necessary.

- Duloxetine (Cymbalta) and milnacipran (Savella) are two antidepressants that have been approved by the FDA for the treatment of fibromyalgia. They are effective in reducing discomfort and promoting relaxation and rest.

• Pregabalin (Lyrica) and gabapentin (Neurontin) are two anticonvulsants commonly recommended for nerve pain and other symptoms of nerve damage.

• Some people find relief from muscle spasms and related discomfort with the use of muscle relaxants.

Therapies:

• To reduce pain and enhance mobility, flexibility, and strength, physical therapists create individualized exercise plans for their patients.

• Occupational therapists can assist people with fibromyalgia in creating plans to deal with everyday tasks and lessen the likelihood of overexertion.

• CBT, or cognitive behavioral therapy, is a form of talk therapy that has been shown to be effective in helping people with fibromyalgia deal with pain, stress, and poor sleep and mood.

• Stress responses like tight muscles and an elevated heart rate can be managed with the use of biofeedback therapy.

• Some people experience relief from pain and enhanced well-being through acupuncture.

• For some people with fibromyalgia, massage therapy is an effective treatment for reducing muscle tension and pain.

Developing a specific treatment strategy for fibromyalgia requires close collaboration with a healthcare provider. To better manage your unique symptoms and enhance your quality of life, your treatment plan may incorporate more than one of the aforementioned medications, therapies, and lifestyle changes.

In order to monitor your progress and make any required adjustments to your treatment plan, it is crucial that you keep all of your follow-up appointments and communicate openly with your healthcare team.

Conclusion

In addition to widespread pain and discomfort, fibromyalgia is characterized by a wide variety of additional symptoms. Research has pointed to anomalies in pain processing, central sensitization, hereditary factors, and environmental triggers as possible contributors to its development, but the specific etiology is still unknown.

Individuals with fibromyalgia may benefit from a combination of medical and psychological interventions to alleviate their symptoms.

Stress reduction, regular exercise, healthy eating, plenty of restful sleep, and a positive social network are all important in the treatment of fibromyalgia.

In order to lessen the severity of the symptoms, doctors may give medications such painkillers, antidepressants, and anticonvulsants.

Individuals can learn coping mechanisms and boost their well-being with the support of therapies including physical therapy, cognitive-behavioral therapy, and biofeedback.

Remember that fibromyalgia is unique to each individual, and that finding the best treatment plan may take time and consistent dialogue with medical professionals.

Many people with fibromyalgia can benefit from enhanced symptom management, enhanced quality of life, and enhanced sense of well-being with the correct approach. Seek the advice of a healthcare practitioner who specializes in fibromyalgia treatment if you or someone you know has been diagnosed with the ailment.

THE END

www.ingramcontent.com/pod-product-compliance
Lightning Source LLC
Chambersburg PA
CBHW060812260726

48660CB00002B/901

9798864980484